Basil Essential Oil

Benefits, Properties, Applications, Studies & Recipes

by Ann Sullivan

Published in USA by:

Ann Sullivan
217 N. Seacrest Blvd #9
Boynton Beach
FL 33425

© Copyright 2017

ISBN-13: ISBN-13: 978-1546634232
ISBN-10: 1546634231

Table of Contents

Introduction

What are essential oils, and how might they be used for therapeutic purposes?

Essential oils are ultra-potent oils, extracted from plants and flowers that have been utilized in medicine for centuries. Presently, they're most commonly used to supplement pharmaceutical medication, but they can also be an effective supplement to pharmaceuticals in the event that you don't have access to them. Before you dismiss essential oils as a means to support the body's natural defenses against injuries and illness, take a look at the historical evidence of the oils' therapeutic competence in practice. Your average age-old medical text will demonstrate that essential oils, herbs, and plenty of other natural ingredients have, for thousands of years, successfully enhanced immune function to meet and defeat any number of ailments and injuries. Though traditional medicine is considered "alternative" now, it was once the gold standard. And, frankly, perhaps it still should be, as these natural age-tested remedies can fortify the body's battlements against everything from simple maladies, like headaches, cuts and bruises, to serious diseases, like cancer.

Essential oils are deemed "essential," because the oils are composed of the "essence" of the plant. The difference between essential oils and other oils – like olive oil or vegetable oil, for instance – is that essential oils have high volatility and reduced fixation, which results in faster evaporation, enabling their popular use in aromatherapy. Even at high temperatures, olive and vegetable oils don't evaporate.

Essential oils are especially necessary when it comes to a major natural or man-made disaster or some potential viral outbreak. In these types of dire situations, you may not have quick access (or any access at all) to your standard pharmaceutical supply; so essential oils, along with other alternative remedies, will be your go-to wellness aids in the case of social collapse, viral outbreak or devastating natural disaster. When medical access is null and void, supplements to our modern-day standard are the only chance we have to keep pathogens at bay.

You probably don't realize that you already use essential oils every day. They're in perfumes, shampoos, soaps, ointments...they're even used in furniture polish. Why are they found in so many aromatic products? Well, basically, because essential oils are super concentrated aromatic liquids, so their scent is remarkably strong. Let's put this into perspective: to steam tea, you use a few leaves of peppermint or juniper; to produce a single ounce of essential oil, five whole *pounds* of peppermint or juniper leaves are required. Some sources claim that to produce twelve pounds of essential oil would necessitate an acre of peppermint, juniper, or any other oil you're looking to produce en masse. Unlike vegetable oil, you don't often find concentrated therapeutic-grade essential oils sold in bulk; instead the oils are often sold in easily carried small, dark bottles, perfect for your GOOD bag (Get Out Of Dodge).

Which is exactly what this book is aiming to help you do – get out of dodge with your most vital of essential oils intact, in particular a good supply of basil essential oil.

Why basil, you ask? Well, in order to get you quickly up to speed on this most essential of oils, below we've provided a condensed synopsis of basil, after which we'll outline in greater detail the oil's history, properties, and common therapeutic uses, so that you – the consumer – might have a better understanding of the oil's benefits and applications. We've even provided supportive remedies for pure basil, as well as blended recipes that incorporate the valuable oil. Chapter 3 will further detail past scientific research on basil essential oil.

Now, let's get down to it – **Essential Oil 101: the Basics of Basil.**

Summary: Basil, or Ocimum basilcum, has therapeutic roots spanning centuries, based largely in the treatment of digestive and respiratory issues, snake bites and fevers. In the 1500s, powdered basil leaves were used as an inhalant to treat chest infections and migraines.

When choosing your basil essential oil, it is important to know that there are dozens of variations of the Basil species and seven specific chemotypes. As these different species have grown in different climates, the chemical properties of each chemotype have been altered. In possessing different properties, each chemotype of basil can be used for different treatments. These chemotypes are listed below.

- Ocimum basilcum CT linol – this chemotype can be used as an antiflatulent or to tone muscles. It also helps fortify the liver and can help treat coronary weakness or depression.
- Ocimum basilcum CT methyl chavicol/estagole CT – this chemotype possesses antispasmodic properties.
- Ocimum basilcum CT eugenol – this chemotype can be applied topically to treat pain or inflammation.
- Ocimum basilcum CT fenchol – this chemotype possesses neurotonic and antiseptic properties.

Description: Basil oil is commonly extracted through steam distillation. The flowers, buds and leaves are most often used. The oil is clear in color, thin in consistency, and has a medium sweet herbal scent.

Uses: Best known for its anti-inflammatory and antispasmodic properties, basil essential oil is also useful as a muscle relaxant. Whether you need to ease a charley horse, a muscle spasm, or simply wish to tone muscles, basil should be your go-to EO when it comes to muscle maintenance. It also can be used to support the body's natural function against coughs, colds, migraines, bronchitis, exhaustion, flu, flatulence, rheumatism, gout, sinusitis, muscle pain, insect bites, and as an insect repellant. When it comes to mood and emotion, basil oil can help with exhaustion, fatigue, insomnia, depression, concentration, memory and burnout.

Properties: Antispasmodic, anti-inflammatory, antibacterial, antiviral, antiseptic, muscle relaxant, stimulant (liver, digestive, nerves and adrenal cortex), and decongestant (lungs, prostate, veins).

Application: Dilute 1:1 with a carrier oil. You can apply topically, diffuse or use as a dietary supplement.

Safety Precautions: Basil has been approved by the FDA for internal consumption and so can be used as a dietary supplement. However, those who are pregnant or breastfeeding should not use this oil, neither should those with epilepsy or children 18 months and younger. You should also test this oil on your skin before extensive topical use, as it may irritate the skin and require further dilution.

Fun facts: Basil is so named, because it was commonly known to the Greeks as the "king of plants." The Greek word for king is "basileum."

Basil goes way back and is even recorded in the first herbalist book of the middle ages, Hildegard's Medicine Book. Hildegard lived between 1098-1179 in Bingen, and this first neuropath recorded more than 12,000 remedies for diseases and medical issues.

Chapter 1 – Benefits of Basil Essential Oil

Basil oil offers a number of therapeutic benefits; but you may be wondering what these benefits are. In this chapter, we'll take a closer look at the history of basil and its many uses.

Cultivation of Basil

Basil, or Ocimum basilicum, is of the Lamiaceae family and is sometimes called sweet basil or St. Joseph's Wort by English speakers. Native to Southeast Asia, India, New Guinea and China, India first domesticated and cultivated basil over 5,000 years ago. Basil grows annually and is perhaps most popular as a culinary herb in Italian cuisine. In fact, basil is a key herb in many a global cuisine, particularly those of southeast Asia, including Laos, Indonesia, Vietnam, Thailand, Taiwan, and Cambodia. The culinary use of basil is due to its sharp, somewhat sweet scent and seasoning.

The plant loves a hot, dry, sunny climate and, in cold climates– like those of Canada, the U.S. and Northern Europe – grows best in a peat pot beneath glass and later planted outside in early summer, so as not to be killed off by frost. The plant thrives in the climates of Australia, southern Europe and the southern United States and can grow anywhere between 12 and 51 inches tall. Though the leaves of most Basil species are green, certain species have purplish leaves, for instance, the species termed "Purple Delight." In most species, white basil flowers appear in a small spike shape.

As with many herbs, several species and hybrids exist which are all known as "basil." Ocimum basilicum, or sweet basil, is the most common species used in Italian cuisine, while three species often crop up in Asian cuisine – Ocimum thyrsiflora, Ocimum tenuiflorum, and Ocimum O. X citriodorum, most commonly known as Thai basil, holy basil, and lemon basil, respectively.

To propagate basil, one can suspend the stems of cuttings in water for two weeks. Roots will develop, as will flowers at the stem. When the plant has fully flowered, black seeds form in the seed pods, which can be planted the next year. If one wants his plant to continue growing, plucking the leaves from the plant will allow basil to sprout new stems in place of the leaves.

A History of Basil

The origin of the name "basil" is up for interpretation. One source claims that the name is derived from the Greek word for "king," which is "basileus." The Oxford English Dictionary indicates that the herb may have been used in royal medicine or bathing. Another speculation by herbalists, John Gerard and Nicholas Culpeper, draws a correlation between the name in relation to a "basilisk," because it was said that the pain from a scorpion sting could be healed with basil and that basil was "an herb of Mars and under the Scorpion, and therefore called Basilicon." Whatever history lies behind the name, in the culinary world, basil has long been touted as the "king of herbs."

History sees basil as a mainstay in many a cultural ritual. In Mexico, suspending basil in a shop window or doorway is purported to attract good fortune. The health of the plant reflects the health of the business; as the herb grows, so should the business' prosperity. The Portuguese celebrate the holidays of Saint Anthony and Saint John by presenting dwarf bush basil in a pot to a lover, accompanied by a poem. In African folklore, basil was, again, cited to defend against scorpions. In Jewish folklore, the herb was used while fasting to maintain strength and energy. In France, basil was often called "l'herbe royale," the "royal herb." In Hinduism, holy basil is venerated. When a person is dying, the herb is placed into the mouth for a secure journey to God, while in Europe, the herb is put into the dead's hands for their own journey to heaven. The Greek

Orthodox Church uses the herb in holy water, as it is believed that Empress Helena found the herb growing on Christ's cross. Even ancient Greeks and ancient Egyptians thought basil was the passport to heaven; they believed the herb would open the doors to God.

Not all cultures held basil in such high esteem, however. Some European lore saw basil as a Satanic symbol, and the Greeks saw it as a symbol of hatred. A French physician, named Hilarius, suggested that too much of the scent could breed scorpions in the mind...Hilarius quite lives up to his name; the idea is hilarious.

In cooking, the herb is even more prevalent across cultures. Basil is used fresh as the final seasoning in many dishes, because drying it or cooking it saps the herb of its flavor. Italian cuisine uses basil to perfection in its signature sauce, pesto, where it's one of the main ingredients alongside garlic, pine nuts and olive oil. In Asia, soaked basil seeds serve as a gelatinous base used in desserts and drinks, but primarily the herb is used to thicken soups or to fry with chicken. It's Thailand, perhaps, that has found one of the most curious culinary purposes for basil; the Thai people steep basil in milk or cream to create basil-based chocolate or ice cream.

As for basil's therapeutic properties, Ayurveda and Siddha medicine (of India and Tamil, respectively) saw this herb as a key ingredient to support the body's natural function against diabetes, stress and asthma. In recent years, basil essential oil has been studied to identify what compounds the oil possesses that serve to provide it with such a range of therapeutic qualities. Basil has been found to have antimicrobial, antiviral and antioxidant properties which allow the herb to offer a range of support; it's even been shown to be beneficial in supporting the body's natural defenses against cancer.

Chemical Components

In order to generate basil essential oil from the plant, the leaves must be steam distilled. This results in the oil's key chemical components, primary of which are (depending upon the species) eugenol, citral, limonene, camphor, camphene, anethole, citronellol, linalool, myrcene, pinene, terpineol, ocimene, linalyl acetate, fenchyl acetate, 1,8-cineole, methyl eugenol, methyl chavicol, and trans-ocimene.

Main Properties of Basil Essential Oil

Along with the properties previously mentioned in the introduction, basil oil possesses antiviral, antibacterial, antispasmodic, anti-inflammatory, diuretic, disinfectant, and decongestant. With such a versatile range, basil is well equipped to fight off any pathogen in the body's path and is a necessary addition to any essential oils kit.

Basil, as mentioned, is composed of many natural chemicals, among them 1,0-cineole, eugenol, linalool, and bergamotene. These components are what instill the enormously beneficial properties within basil essential oil. We'll outline these properties below.

Disinfectant & Cleaner

As a disinfectant, basil can be added to household cleaners to disinfect your home. As a cleaning agent, basil eliminates contamination, which means your household will be sick less often. Basil can be used to clean dishes, clothing, and practically any surface.

Antioxidant

Anything high in antioxidants – whether fruit, beans, or essential oils – is a powerful advocate for your body. Antioxidants both protect against free radicals and repair their damage. What are free radicals? Free radicals are destructive chemicals that invade your body, produced by substances both inside and out. Some free radicals (or oxidants) form through normal bodily reactions, like inflammation, metabolism and aerobic respiration. Other free radicals form outside the body, but enter it due to exposure. These include harmful pollutants, toxins, smoking, drinking alcohol, X-rays, and UV rays, to name a few. Although our bodies produce their own antioxidants, these often become damaged as we grow older; thus, introducing antioxidants into our bodies via essential oils allows these nutrients and enzymes to assist in chemical reactions which destroy the oxidants or free radicals. Basil essential oil is a moderate antioxidant, aiming to detox the body of free radicals that lead to disease.

Antibacterial

Basil's antibacterial properties make it a powerful protectant against diseases produced by bacteria, such as skin issues and infections. What's great is that, unlike some prescription drugs, basil has no ill effects on body wellness or on the natural flora that exists within the stomach and intestines.

Antiviral

The antiviral protection that basil essential oil grants will empower the immune system at its core, building up a tougher wall of security that most colds, measles or mumps are unlikely to scale. By boosting white blood cell count and function, this immune stimulant will ensure that your body is better prepared to protect against deadly viral infections.

Anti-inflammatory

External or internal inflammation can be reduced

through the use of basil essential oil. For instance, if you or your patient has swollen fingers from arthritis or a swollen knee from a sport's injury, oral application of basil essential oil may decrease irritation or redness, while also soothing the pain that accompanies inflammation.

Antispasmodic

The antispasmodic properties of basil essential oil make it beneficial to such surgical processes as colonoscopy, gastroscopy, and intraluminally-applied double-contrast barium enema.

Diuretic

If you're looking to lose water weight and reduce blood pressure, basil essential oil is your agent. The oil stimulates urination, promoting not only the loss of water weight, but the loss of fats, uric acid, sodium, and other body toxins.

Decongestant

As a decongestant, basil essential oil can alleviate nasal congestion in the upper respiratory tract.

Common Therapeutic Uses

Basil has traditionally been used for its soothing and healing properties and, as an antioxidant, basil essential oil is particularly helpful when it comes to fighting inflammation and bacterial or viral infections. Let's take a look at some of the oil's primary therapeutic uses.

Digestion

As a digestive tonic, basil essential oil's carminative properties serve to support the body's natural function against constipation, flatulence, indigestion, and stomach cramps. Gas is quickly relieved from the stomach and intestines, and the oil's colic properties further help to relieve uncomfortable bowel pain.

Nausea & Vomiting

Basil essential oil can relieve nausea and vomiting from morning sickness, motion sickness, or illness.

Cold & Flu

For those of us who are susceptible to seasonal cold and flu viruses (so...everyone), providing your immune system with a reliable mechanism of defense can mean the difference between illness and wellness. Basil essential oil protects your immune system and relieves fever and cough, which often accompany a cold or flu.

Skin wellness

Basil essential oil can be used both to stave off infections, heal and maintain your skin's wellness. The oil is a topical antiseptic and, as mentioned, has been shown to effectively support the body's natural function against infections in wounds and cuts, as well as in burns and blisters. Basil is also a great antidote for bites and stings of all sorts (remember the scorpion), including bug, bee, and snake. It relieves itching and helps heal the wound. Basil can also be used cosmetically to give dull, lackluster skin and hair an even tone and an attractive glow. It can also support the body's natural function against acne or other unsightly skin infections.

Coughs & Respiratory Infection

The antispasmodic properties of basil essential oil make it a soothing antidote to coughs and other respiratory issues, like bronchitis, asthma, or sinus infection.

Pain Relief

Basil's analgesic qualities make it an effective pain reliever to be used in support the body's natural function againsting headache, sprains, injuries, wounds, scars, bruises, burns, and arthritis. It's a surefire aid to any sports muscle sprain or recovery pain from surgery.

Stress Disorders

Whether it be physical stress or mental stress, basil's fresh aroma, alongside its therapeutic properties, enable its use in easing nerves, anxiety, melancholy, and depression. It can soothe mental fatigue and the associated migraines that come along with mental wellness issues. The oil is said to stimulate clarity and strong mental wellness.

Blood Circulation

Blood circulation and bodily metabolic function is given a boost with the use of basil essential oil.

Safety Precautions & Common Applications

Safety

Some adverse effects may evolve when using pure essential oils. Some essential oils should not be used when pregnant, for example, as they may cause miscarriage. Allergic reactions, too, may occur, especially when applied topically. Always administer an allergy test before committing fully to topical application. When used with other medications, essential oils may react negatively. If you are on any current prescription medications or have a chronic illness, such as high blood pressure, epilepsy or liver disease, then researching the effects of essential oils against your own personal medical history will eliminate any potentially problematic issues.

Basil has been approved by the FDA for internal consumption and so can be used as a dietary supplement. However, ensure that your basil oil is of high-quality, therapeutic grade, or it should not be used for therapeutic treatments. Those who are pregnant or breastfeeding should not use this oil, neither should those with epilepsy or children 18 months and younger. You should also test this oil on your skin before extensive topical use, as it may irritate the skin and require further dilution.

Blends

Oftentimes, essential oils are manufactured as blends of several pure oils. For instance, a mixture of cinnamon, clove, rosemary, and eucalyptus. This blend can be used to boost the immune system to help support the body's defenses against colds, viruses and flus. The downside to blends is that the more oils added to the mix, the higher the probability your patient may react negatively to the blend if he/she is prone to allergies. There is also the possibility of phototoxicity when working with blends.

Regardless of these possible effects, essential oils are a viable option for support the body's defenses againsting a number of conditions. Those looking to enhance the maintenance of their own personal wellness, or that of their families, should become educated on the uses of essential oils, their natural remedies and the methods of application. Only then can you begin building your kit of essential oils for survival.

Chapter 2 – Recipes for Basil Essential Oil

In this chapter, we'll offer various recipes for basil essential oil, both for pure basil treatments and blends. For pure treatments, we've provided the appropriate application and dosage to treat specific ailments, from acne to sinus infections. When it comes to blends, herbalists and aromatherapists often combine basil essential oil with bergamot, clary sage, clove bud, geranium, lime, lemon, hyssop, juniper, eucalyptus, neroli, marjoram, rosemary, melissa and lavender. We'll offer some fantastic supportive blending options in the second half of this chapter.

Pure Supportive Remedies

Addiction

To help alleviate addiction, dilute basil essential oil in a

1:1 ratio with a carrier oil and apply topically, massaging over the solar plexus and the heart. You can also administer aromatically, diffusing throughout the home or inhaling directly from the bottle.

Adrenal Fatigue

Combat adrenal fatigue by diffusing basil essential oil or adding a few drops to your bathwater. You can also dilute a drop of basil to every three drops of carrier oil and massage into the feet or over the adrenals every night.

Amenorrhea

Amenorrhea, or skipping a menstrual cycle, can be avoided by diluting basil essential oil in a 1:1 ratio with a carrier oil and applying topically over the lower abdomen, as well as into the ankles and the soles of the feet.

Anxiety

To relieve anxiety, place one drop of basil essential oil into your palm and rub your hands together. Place your hand over your nose and mouth and inhale. You can also diffuse throughout your home to relieve tension and stress.

Autism

Basil can help provide emotional balance in autistic children, while at the same time, emphasizing the positive end of the strong emotional spectrum. To apply, dilute 1 drop of basil essential oil to every 3 drops of a carrier oil and apply topically, massaging into the feet each night.

Bronchitis

Ease bronchitis by diluting basil essential oil in a 1:1 ratio with a carrier oil, then apply topically, massaging into the throat, chest and back. Additionally, you can steam two drops of basil essential oil in a pan of water, remove the steaming pan from the stove, pour into a bowl, place a towel over your head and inhale. You can also diffuse throughout the room, place a drop of oil onto your shirt collar, or inhale directly for effective easement throughout the day.

Bursitis

To help alleviate the pain and inflammation of bursitis, dilute basil essential oil in a 1:1 ratio with a carrier oil, then apply topically, massaging into the affected area.

Carpal Tunnel Syndrome

Carpal tunnel syndrome can be eased by by diluting basil essential oil in a 1:1 ratio with a carrier oil, then apply topically, massaging into the affected area toward the shoulder, while placing a good amount of pressure against the muscles and tendons.

Chronic Fatigue

To combat chronic fatigue, place a few drops of basil essential oil into your bathwater, diffuse throughout the home, or dilute the oil in a 1:1 ratio with a carrier oil and massage into the soles of the feet.

Cuts

To accelerate skin repair, stave off infection, and soothe pain, dilute basil essential oil in a 1:1 ratio with a carrier oil and apply topically to the affected area.

Earache

Relieve earaches or infections by diluting 1 drop of basil oil to 3 drops of carrier oil and apply topically over and behind the ear, but not within it.

Fear

To help eliminate unwarranted fear, dilute basil essential oil in a 1:1 ratio with a carrier oil and apply topically, massaging over the solar plexus and the heart. You can also administer aromatically, diffusing throughout the home or inhaling directly from the bottle.

Hernia

Hernias can be targeted with basil essential oil by diluting in a 1:1 ratio with a carrier oil and apply topically, massaging gently over the affected area.

Infertility

Stimulate fertility by diluting basil essential oil in a 1:1 ratio with a carrier oil and apply topically, massaging over the reproductive organs and into the reflex points of the feet. You can also diffuse throughout the room for a similar effect.

Insect Bites/Stings

Dilute basil essential oil in a 1:3 ratio with a carrier oil and apply to the affected area to protect against infections and eliminate irritation. Apply up to three times daily.

Labor

When transitioning into labor, dilute basil essential oil in a 1:1 ratio with a carrier oil and massage into the reflex points of the feet and into the lower back.

Lactation (Increasing)

Increase lactation by diluting basil essential oil in a 1:1 ratio with a carrier oil and apply topically, massaging into the breasts toward the lymph nodes (underarms) twice daily.

Loss of Smell

To stimulate the sense of smell, diffuse basil essential oil throughout the home or inhale directly from the bottle. You can also dilute the oil in a 1:1 ratio with a carrier oil and apply topically over the sinuses and into the reflex points of the feet.

Lymphatic System Cleanse

To cleanse the lymphatic system, basil essential oil can be applied topically without dilution (if your skin is not sensitive) to induce sweating.

Mental Fatigue

To combat mental fatigue, place a few drops of basil

essential oil into your bathwater, or dilute in a 1:1 ratio with a carrier oil and massage into your chest, scalp, and into the soles of the feet. You can also diffuse throughout the home.

Menstrual Cramps

Relieve menstrual cramps by applying basil essential oil topically. Massage into the lower abdomen and back and into the reflex points of the feet.

Migraines

Migraines can be relieved with basil oil to relieve pain. Diffuse throughout the room or, for a more direct application, dilute basil essential oil in a 1:1 ratio with a carrier oil and apply topically over the area of pain, into the temples and the base of the neck. Avoid the eyes.

Mouth Ulcers

Support the body's natural defenses against mouth ulcers by placing a drop in a glass of water and rinsing the mouth three times daily.

Muscle Spasms

To relieve muscle spasms, dilute basil essential oil in a 1:1 ratio with a carrier oil and massage the solution into the affected area, toward the heart.

Muscular Dystrophy

Muscular dystrophy can be alleviated by diluting basil essential oil in a 1:1 ratio with a carrier oil and massaging the solution in a full-body massage and into the reflex points of the feet.

Nervousness

Nervousness can be calmed through directly inhaling basil essential oil. Pour a drop into your hands, rub your palms together, cup them over your nose, and breathe deeply in and out for several minutes.

Oily Hair

Eliminate oily or greasy hair by placing a drop of basil essential oil in your shampoo and using as normal.

Ovarian Cyst

Support the body's natural function against an ovarian cyst by diluting basil essential oil in a 1:1 ratio with a carrier oil and apply topically, massaging over the area of the ovaries twice daily. You can also diffuse or steam two drops of basil essential oil in a pan of water. Then remove the steaming pan from the stove, pour into a bowl, place a towel over your head and inhale.

Schmidt's Syndrome

Ease Schmidt's Syndrome by diluting basil essential oil in a 1:1 ratio with a carrier oil and apply topically, massaging the oil into the reflex points of the feet.

Snake/Spider Bites

For snake or spider bites, dilute basil essential oil in a 1:1 ratio with a carrier oil and apply gently to the affected area to protect against infections and eliminate irritation.

Apply up to three times daily.

Viral Hepatitis

Support the body's natural defenses against hepatitis by diffusing or steaming two drops of basil essential oil in a pan of water. Then remove the steaming pan from the stove, pour into a bowl, place a towel over your head and inhale. If you don't feel it's done its job the first time, you can reheat that same water and use it once more without adding more oil. You can also dilute basil in a 1:1 ratio with a carrier oil and apply topically, massaging over the body and into the soles of the feet every day.

Wounds

Enhance wound healing by adding a few drops of basil essential oil to into a spray bottle filled with distilled water. Spray over the wound. You may also apply a few drops to a spritz bath and soak wound for 10-15 minutes. You can also dilute basil in a 1:1 ratio with a carrier oil and apply to the affected area.

Blends

Anti-Anxiety Bath

Ingredients

- 2 drops Basil Essential Oil
- 2 drops Grapefruit Essential Oil
- 2 drops Geranium Essential Oil
- 3 drops Lavender Essential Oil
- 3 drops Ylang Ylang Essential Oil

Directions

To wind down, de-stress, and combat anxiety, add all ingredients to your bathwater and stir to disperse. Then inhale deeply while you soak for 20 minutes, but avoid getting water in your eyes, as it may sting.

Arthritis

Ingredients

- 1 drop Sage Essential Oil
- 1 drop Basil Essential Oil
- 1 drop Cinnamon Essential Oil
- 4 drops Sweet Almond Oil

Directions

To combat arthritis or sore muscles, combine all ingredients, blending well, and massage into affected area.

Bug Repellent

Ingredients

- 1 cup 190-Proof Grain Alcohol
- 20 drops Basil Essential Oil
- 2 cups Water

Directions

For a potent bug spray, combine all ingredients in a spray bottle and shake well. Spray on your skin, into entrances and window sills, and all around you, shaking well before each use.

Charley Horse

Ingredients

- 4 drops Basil Essential Oil
- 2 drops Marjoram Essential Oil
- 2 drops Lemongrass Essential Oil
- 6 drops Coconut Oil

Directions

To relieve Charley Horses or other cramps, place all ingredients into a small bowl or container and blend thoroughly then administer topically, massaging into the affected area.

Detoxification

Ingredients

- 2 drops Juniper Essential Oil
- 2 drops Lavender Essential Oil
- 2 drops Grapefruit Essential Oil
- 2 drops Basil Essential Oil
- 2 drops Cypress Essential Oil
- 30 mL Carrier Oil

Directions

To flush out toxins and boost circulation, combine all ingredients, blending well, and massage into the reflex points in the feet.

Diabetes

Ingredients

- 2 drops Basil Essential Oil
- 3 drops Coriander Essential Oil
- 1 tsp Carrier Oil

Directions

Apply topically to the reflex points in the feet and to the back of the neck and under the tongue two times a day.

Earache

Ingredients

- 1 drop Basil Essential Oil
- 1 drop Geranium Essential Oil
- 2 drops Carrier Oil

Directions

To relieve the pain from earaches, combine all ingredients and apply on the ear's surface, as well as behind the ear. You can also add a drop of each oil to a cotton ball to be placed over the ear canal, but do not press inside the ear.

Exam Energizer

Ingredients

- 3 drops Oregano Essential Oil
- 5 drops Melaleuca Essential Oil
- 5 drops Lemon Essential Oil

Directions

To get your head in the game for an exam, place 1-2 drops of basil essential oil on your shirt collar or a small cloth and inhale before and during your exam. Basil will provide clarity and concentration.

Fatigue

Ingredients

- 4 drops Rosemary Essential Oil
- 2 drops Basil Essential Oil
- 30 mL Carrier Oil

Directions

To combat tiredness and exhaustion, combine all ingredients, blending well, and massage into the reflex points in the feet.

Fungal Infections

Ingredients

- 3 drops Grapefruit Essential Oil
- 2 drops Cinnamon Essential Oil
- 1 drop Basil Essential Oil
- 1 drop Patchouli Essential Oil
- ½ ounce Carrier Oil

Directions

To eliminate fungal infections, combine all ingredients and apply topically to affected area.

Hepatitis

Ingredients

- 4 drops Basil Essential Oil
- 4 drops Myrrh Essential Oil
- 4 drops Cypress Essential Oil
- 8 drops Coconut Oil

Directions

To support the body's natural defenses against hepatitis, place all ingredients into a small bowl or container and blend thoroughly then administer topically, massaging into the liver and into the reflex points of the hands and feet.

You can also place 2 drops of each essential oil into a "00" capsule, and ingest 1 capsule twice daily.

Mental Stimulant Bath

Ingredients

- 2 drops Rosemary Essential Oil
- 4 drops Basil Essential Oil
- 4 drops Lemon Essential Oil
- 1 Tbsp Grapeseed Oil

Directions

To stimulate and energize your mind, add all ingredients to your bathwater and stir to disperse. Then inhale deeply while you soak for 20 minutes, but avoid getting water in your eyes, as it may sting.

Menstrual Cramps

Ingredients

- 3 drops Basil Essential Oil
- 3 drops Clary Sage Essential Oil
- 3 drops Coconut Oil

Directions

To relieve menstrual cramps, place all ingredients into a small bowl or container and blend thoroughly then administer topically, massaging into the abdomen every hour until pain is eliminated. Drink water for added support.

Migraines

Ingredients

- 4 drops Basil Essential Oil
- 3 drops Marjoram Essential Oil
- 3 drops Ylang Ylang Essential Oil
- 6 drops Coconut Oil

Directions

To enhance the body's natural defenses against migraines or headaches, combine all ingredients in a small bowl or jar and blend well. Then administer topically, massaging the solution into the temples, forehead, the shoulders and the back of the neck.

Spider Bites

Ingredients

- 3 drops Basil Essential Oil
- 3 drops Lemon Essential Oil
- 4 ounces Distilled Water

Directions

To strengthen the body's natural defenses against spider bites, place all ingredients into a spray bottle and shake thoroughly then administer topically, spraying onto the affected area.

Stings (Bees, Wasps, Hornets)

Ingredients

- 4 drops Lavender Essential Oil
- 2 drops Basil Essential Oil
- 4 drops Carrier Oil
- 4 ounces Distilled Water

Directions

Combine all ingredients in a spray bottle and spray directly to the sting site every 30 minutes.

Study Blend

Ingredients

- 2 drops Rosemary Essential Oil
- 3 drops Basil Essential Oil
- 5 drops Lemon Essential Oil
- ½ tsp Carrier Oil

Directions

In a small container combine all ingredients and blend well. Apply to the wrists or diffuse.

Uplifting Massage Blend

Ingredients

- 20 mL Carrier Oil
- 3 drops Bergamot Essential Oil
- 3 drops Rosemary Essential Oil
- 3 drops Eucalyptus Essential Oil
- 3 drops Lime Essential Oil
- 3 drops Basil Essential Oil
- 5 drops Spearmint Essential Oil

Directions

For an uplifting massage, combine all oils in a small glass jar or container, cap with the lid, and shake until well blended. Use as normal.

Chapter 3 – Basil Essential Oil Studies

Many studies have been done on essential oils to uncover and prove their therapeutic qualities. In the case of the great number of basil studies, many of the properties attributed to the essential oil (noted in this book and elsewhere) are quite often validated through scientific research from accredited universities and published by reputable scientific journals. In this chapter, we'll discuss a small portion of these studies. It's important to note that research on essential oils is constant and evolving. Keep abreast with any recent research, as it may turn up even further valuable uses of these miracle oils.

Study 1 – Cytotoxic

In this study published by *Food Science and Nutrition*, the antimicrobial, antioxidant and cytotoxic properties of many essential oils were examined, with the following results: "Chemical composition, antioxidant, antimicrobial and cytotoxic activities of...Ocimum basilicum (OB) essential oil (OBO) were examined...(it) could be used as an effective source of natural antioxidant and antibacterial additive to protect foods from oxidative damages and foodborne pathogens. Furthermore, (ocimum basilicum) could be promising candidate for antitumor drug design."

When the cell line is broached by an essential oil, the result is cell death, which makes the oil "cytotoxic" and, thus, a potential antitumoral candidate. This study revealed basil essential oil's potential use as an antitumor drug, and as a natural food preservative. Due to its antibacterial and antioxidant properties, basil essential oil could increase a product's shelf-life, as well as improve the chances of safe consumption.

Reference
http://www.ncbi.nlm.nih.gov/pubmed/24804073

http://www.ncbi.nlm.nih.gov/pmc/articles/PMC3959961/pdf/fsn30002-0146.pdf

Study 2 – Antimalarial

In this study published by *Parasite*, the antimicrobial effects of basil essential oil were examined, with the following results: "The biological activities of essential oils from three plants grown in Cameroon: Ocimum basilicum, Ocimum canum, and Cymbopogon citratus were tested against Plasmodium falciparum and mature-stage larvae of Anopheles funestus...These essential oils can be recommended for the development of natural biocides for fighting the larvae of malaria vectors and for the isolation of natural products with anti-malarial activity."

Plasmodium falciparum and Anopheles funestus are malaria-causing parasites, transmitted by the Anopheles mosquito. This particular species results in the most lethal form of malaria, with the highest mortality rates and the most complications in treatment. Most of the global malarial infections are in Africa, with over 247 million human infections to date, worldwide, 98% of which come out of Africa. 75% of these African malarial cases are caused by this species, P. falciparum, which causes nearly all malarial deaths, with the other strains of malaria being much easier to manage. Malarial symptoms include, nausea and vomiting, fatigue, headache, chills, sweats, and fever.

This study showed that, while C. citratus was the most active against both P. falciparum and A. funestus, both O. canum and O. basilicum showed aggressive activity against the parasites as well, with basil essential oil turning out an IC50 value (50% inhibition in vitro) of 21 ± 4.6 μg/mL.

Consequently, the study indicates that basil essential oil can serve as a natural biocide in anti-malarial products and in combatting the larvae of malaria-carrying mosquitoes.

Reference
http://www.ncbi.nlm.nih.gov/pubmed/24995776

http://www.ncbi.nlm.nih.gov/pmc/articles/PMC4082313/pdf/parasite-21-33.pdf

Study 3 – Hep C Antiviral

In this study published by the *Brazilian Journal of Microbiology*, the antiviral effects of basil essential oil were examined, with the following results: "The bovine viral diarrhoea virus (BVDV) is suggested as a model for antiviral studies of the hepatitis C virus (HCV). The antiviral activity of the essential oil of Ocimum basilicum and the monoterpenes camphor, thymol and 1,8-cineole against BVDV was investigated...The higher activities achieved by the monoterpenes in the virucidal assay suggest that these compounds act directly on the viral particle."

Proven in 1989, the infectious disease, hepatitis C, is spread through the blood via intravenous drug use, transfusions, or unsterilized medical equipment. Affecting an estimated 150 million people globally, the disease most often impacts the liver and can lead to liver scarring or cirrhosis of the liver. The asymptomatic infection can move from acute to chronic after several years, with those experiencing cirrhosis of the liver ultimately facing potentially fatal health issues, like esophageal and gastric varices, liver cancer or liver failure.

In its early stages acute symptoms are generally mild and include weight loss, decreased appetite, muscle and joint pain, nausea and fatigue. Chronic infection occurs in around 80% of those infected, with most individuals experiencing few or no symptoms within the first couple decades after becoming infected.

This study examined the effects of basil essential oil and its cytotoxic compounds against bovine viral diarrhoea virus, which is often used in scientific research as an equivalent to hep C. In the study, two of basil essential oil's chemical components, 1,8-cineole and camphor demonstrated the lowest cytotoxicities and the best antiviral activities, with 1,8-cineol SI = 9.05 and camphor SI = 13.88 (SI stands for the Système Internationale or the International System of scientific measurements). The study demonstrates basil essential oil's general antiviral properties, as well as its potential in targeted treatment of hep C.

Reference

http://www.ncbi.nlm.nih.gov/pubmed/24948933

http://www.ncbi.nlm.nih.gov/pmc/articles/PMC4059298/pdf/bjm-45-209.pdf]

Study 4 – Antibacterial

In this study published by *Molecules,* the antibacterial effects of basil essential oil were examined, with the following results: "The considerable therapeutical problems of persistent infections caused by multidrug-resistant bacterial strains constitute a continuing need to find effective antimicrobial agents. The aim of this study was to demonstrate the activities of basil (Ocimum basilicum L.) and rosemary (Rosmarinus officinalis L.) essential oils against multidrug- resistant clinical strains of Escherichia coli...The results showed that both tested essential oils are active against all of the clinical strains from Escherichia coli including extended-spectrum β-lactamase positive bacteria, but basil oil possesses a higher ability to inhibit growth. These studies may hasten the application of essential oils in the treatment and prevention of emergent resistant strains in nosocomial infections."

Escherichia coli is a Gram-positive bacterium that can result in serious food poisoning. After a detailed analysis, this study showed that basil essential oil demonstrated inhibitory activity against several strains of Escherichia coli obtained from patients with respiratory tract and urinary tract infections, as well as infections of the skin and abdomen and from hospital equipment. Included in the testing was the main strain, ATCC 25922. Basil essential oil showed high inhibition against the strains and furthermore in bacterial growth, indicating that the oil can be used to stave off and strengthen the body's natural defenses against

E. coli.

Reference
http://www.ncbi.nlm.nih.gov/pubmed/23921795]

http://www.mdpi.com/1420-3049/18/8/9334]

Study 5 – Leishmaniasis

In this study published by the *Tehran University of Medical Sciences Publication*, the antibacterial effects of basil essential oil were examined, with the following results: "The leishmanicidal and cytotoxic activity of ten essential oils obtained from ten plant specimens were evaluated...Cytotoxicity was tested on J774 macrophages and leishmanicidal activity was assessed against four species of Leishmania associated with cutaneous leishmaniasis...The essential oil of Ocimum basilicum was active against promastigotes of Leishmania and innocuous to J774 macrophages at concentrations up to 1600 μg/mL and should be further investigated for leishmanicidal activity in others in vitro and in vivo experimental models."

Cutaneous leishmaniasis is the most common form of a skin infection transmitted by sandflies which carry the single-celled parasite which causes Leishmania. Around 20 species of Leishmania-causing cutaneous leishmaniasis are in known existence. Cutaneous leishmaniasis results in red lesions from the bug bite which are raised from the skin. Eventually, the lesion ulcerates and bacterial infection occurs. Two types of cutaneous leishmaniasis are post kala-azar dermal leishmaniasis (PKDL) and mucocutaneous leishmaniasis. PKDL can recur in the skin of diagnosed individuals for up to 20 years after partial or adequate treatment. The most destructive form of cutaneous leishmaniasis is mucocutaneous leishmaniasis. The lesions produced by this form of the infection can disfigure and destroy the face.

This study analyzed seven essential oils against Leishmania parasites. Five of the oils were toxic against J774 macrophages, and basil essential oil was found to be highly active against promastigotes (a common morphology in the insect host) of Leishmania.

Reference

http://www.ncbi.nlm.nih.gov/pubmed/23682270

http://www.ncbi.nlm.nih.gov/pmc/articles/PMC3655250/pdf/IJPA-8-129.pdf]

Study 6 – Acne

In this study published by *Biomedica*, the antibacterial effects of basil essential oil on acne were examined, with the following results: "Currently, the antimicrobial resistance has developed in bacterial strains involved in the development of acne. Therefore, alternatives to antibiotic treatment have become necessary...Gel formulations were designed based on essential oils and acetic acid, and their effectiveness was evaluated in patients affected by acne...All groups reported an improvement of the acne condition, which ranged between 43% and 75% clearance of lesions. Evidence of treatment disappeared within minutes, showing little discomfort or side effects after application."

The study examined essential oils as potential acne treatments, and basil essential oil was among those tested. The treatment followed 28 patients, divided into groups of four. Each group applied gel treatments composed of various combinations, including a pure essential oil treatment, a treatment of essential oils combined with acetic acid, keratolytic medicine, and a combo of acetic acid and kerolytic medicine. Each week, the patient's' skin was checked, during which it was discovered that the essential oil application was chemically and physically stable throughout the course of treatment. All applications proved to treat acne, resulting in anywhere from 43%-75% clearance of the condition.

Reference

http://www.ncbi.nlm.nih.gov/pubmed/23235794]

http://www.scielo.org.co/scielo.php?script=sci_pdf&pid=S0120-41572012000100014&lng=en&nrm=iso&tlng=es]

Study 7 – Antibacterial

In this study published by *Biosci. Biotechnol. Biochem.*, the effects basil essential oil has on head lice were examined, with the following results: "Nine essential oils were examined for antimicrobial activity against reference and clinical strains of Salmonella Enteritidis. Based on the size of the inhibition zone and the minimal inhibitory concentration, basil oil had the strongest antimicrobial activity against all the tested bacteria, and S. Enteritidis SE3 was the most sensitive strain to all the tested oils...The results from this study confirm the potential use of basil oil as an antimicrobial agent to control S. Enteritidis in food."

In summary, this study showed that basil essential oil was incredibly effective as an antibacterial agent against pathogenic strains of Salmonella entericidis, which most commonly infects cattle, poultry, and other animals. It can also be spread to humans, however; particularly vulnerable are those who work closely with animals playing host to the bacteria. S. entericidis can also cause infection through contaminated raw chicken eggs, which are often used in homemade foods, like cookies, cakes, or mayonnaise and can therefore infect those who consume these goods. Basil essential oil was able to eradicate this bacteria, due primarily to its chemical constituents, linalool, 1,8-cineole, and eugenol, demonstrating its potential as an antimicrobial agent in food.

Reference
http://www.ncbi.nlm.nih.gov/pubmed/20530897]

https://www.jstage.jst.go.jp/article/bbb/74/6/74_90939/pdf]

Study 8 – Ear Infection

In this study published by the *Journal of Infectious Disease*, the antimicrobial effects of basil essential oil were examined, with the following results: "Essential oils are volatile and can have good antimicrobial activity. We compared the effects of oil of basil (Ocimum basilicum) and essential oil components (thymol, carvacrol, and salicylaldehyde) to those of a placebo when placed in the ear canal of rats with experimental acute otitis media caused by pneumococci or Haemophilus influenzae...Essential oils or their components placed in the ear canal can provide effective treatment of acute otitis media."

This study tested basil essential oil against acute otitis media caused by pneumococci or Haemophilus influenzae. Otitis media is a common childhood inflammation of the middle ear, although it can occur well into adulthood. Acute otitis media often results in ear pain, which has the potential to become chronic. The otitis media tested in this study was resultant of pneumococci or Haemophilus influenzae. Pneumococci is a Gram-positive strain of the pathogenic bacterium, Streptococcus pneumoniae, which causes – you guessed it! – pneumonia, along with a number of other infectious diseases, such as rhinitis, bronchitis, conjunctivitis, and endocarditis, just to name a few. Pneumonia infects the sinuses, nasal cavity and the respiratory tract and, moreover, can cause meningitis in immunocompromised individuals, like children and the elderly.

Haemophilus influenzae is a Gram-negative bacterium of the Pasteurellaceae family. Mistakenly believed to result in influenza, this bacterium was termed "bacterial influenza" up until 1933, when influenza was found to be viral. However, though not the culprit for influenza, H. influenzae is no innocent; it can cause a whole litany of localized and invasive infections. So prominent is H.influenzae in the world of science and health that, in 1995, it became the first free-living organism to have its entire genome sequenced.

With such health stakes as these two bacterial strains present, as can be assumed, an antidote to the acute otitis media resulting from these strains is vital to the treatment of diseases caused by pneumococci or Haemophilus influenzae. Basil essential showed exceptional antimicrobial activity at minimum inhibitory levels against both strains – 6%-75% of rats infected with pneumococci were cured, and 56%-81% of rats infected with H. Influenzae – and can therefore serve as an effective treatment for acute otitis.

Reference
http://www.ncbi.nlm.nih.gov/pubmed/15871121]

http://jid.oxfordjournals.org/content/191/11/1876.full.pdf+html]

Chapter 4 – The Ins & Outs of Essential Oils

Where do essential oils come from?

Plants and plant species naturally produce essential oils for various reasons, one being to draw pollinator insects to them, another being to repel invading organisms (bacteria, animals). A number of chemical compounds compose each plant's essential oil, and the combination of these compounds is specific to each oil, which then instills in the oil its own unique properties. Essential oils can be harnessed from all sorts of plant components, including flowers, leaves, bark, fruit, roots, and resin. For instance, cinnamon oil is harnessed from bark, lemon oil from the peel, and lavender oil from lavender flowers. Certain plants can produce a few chemical variants of the same essential oil, which are acquired from different parts of the plant.

Some of these parts produce a large amount of oil, while others produce just a smidgen. The oil's quality and potency depends upon a number of factors, including the subspecies of the plant, its soil conditions, the time of year and even the time of day you harvest it.

How are essential oils extracted?

Essential oils can be extracted from plants through various methods, including pressing, distillation, solvent and maceration. Let's take a brief look at each:

Pressing Method

Commonly used with citrus fruit, the pressing method extracts the oil through a technique which involves pushing the fruit peels through a press. Oily fruits and plants are best suited for this technique. Orange oil, for example, is extracted from orange skins through the pressing method.

Distillation Method

This technique harkens back to the days of old-timey moonshiners, as the same sort of method used to create strong liquor can be used to extract essential oils. Using a still, boiled water and plant materials will create steam which is then cooled by coils and condensed into a combination of water and oil. This combination doesn't mix, so the oil can then be extracted from it.

Solvent Method

Through a multi-step process, certain plant and flower

oils can be extracted using alcohol and other solvents, which extort the essential oil from the plant materials.

Maceration Method

When a "carrier" or fixed oil or lard is mixed with the plant material and set out in the sun, over a period of time, the carrier oil is infused with the plant's essence. Heat sources, other than the sun, are often used to speed the process. Throughout the process, more plant material is added to produce a more potent oil.

How do you use essential oils?

Although some studies about the effectiveness of essential oils are conducted by small companies or even individuals, a number of them are conducted by the food and cosmetic industries. In general, the pharmaceutical industry shows next to no interest in herbal remedies, primarily because there are few options to patent such products. Being as such, the product's lack of profitability results in a lack of research funding. Regardless, the historical uses of essential oils tell us what we need to know: these oils have been effectively administered for centuries. The therapeutic qualifications of essential oils can be plotted in the survival of the human race across cultures and generations.

Another reason that studies on essential oils have not resulted in much conclusive evidence as to their overall effectiveness is because definitive results are sometimes difficult to prove, as the quality of each batch of oil can vary for a number of reasons. One is that essential oils are impossible to standardize. As mentioned above, even the slightest variance in soil conditions and the time of harvesting – as well as innumerable other factors – will produce a different product quality and potency. In addition, essential oils are often obtained from various species of the same plant; Eucalyptus radiata and Eucalyptus globulus can both be used in the making of therapeutic-grade eucalyptus oil and, as a result, they may have slightly different properties and degrees of strength or effectiveness.

Just as there are a number of methods by which to extract essential oils, there are a number of methods to administer them therapeutically. The variety of chemical compounds in each essential oil means that their benefits and applications also vary across the board. Below are a few of these methods.

Topical Administration

Direct application of many essential oils works like a sponge, as skin sops up chemicals and other things (like sunlight, for instance). Topical application is best when you want to clear up an ailment on the skin's surface or in the underlying muscle tissue. When applying topically, you may either massage the oil into the skin or simply dab on the skin for therapeutic results. You might combine the essential oil with a carrier oil for topical use in order to dilute its potency. This is safer, as the oil is so concentrated. You may support your body's defenses against rash or muscle pain in this manner, but you should always test your patient for allergies before applying. Adverse effects are produced by natural chemicals as much as synthetic ones; poison ivy, for example.

To test for allergens, place a drop or two on your patient's inner forearm. If a rash develops within 12 to 24 hours, then the patient is allergic. In addition, phototoxicity – sun exposure resulting in an exacerbated burn – may be an issue when citrus oils are applied topically. So one must proceed with caution when applying essential oils using this method.

Inhalation Therapy

Commonly known as "aromatherapy", this essential oil application is effective for inner ailments, like sore throat or cold. In a steaming bowl of distilled or sterilized water, add a few drops of essential oil and, with a towel over your head, bend over the bowl and inhale. The towel captures the vapors, making the technique even more effective. Essential oils can also be placed in a diffuser or potpourri throughout a room to produce somewhat diluted therapeutic effects.

Ingestion

When using this method, proceed with caution. Direct ingestion of essential oils must be monitored and applied in small doses that are diluted in a tablespoon or more of any carrier oil – olive oil, for example. If you are unsure of dosage amounts, make a tea with the relevant herb instead. Although the effects of this diluted use may be weaker, this application is a better alternative than an overdose of essential oils.

What are the general benefits of using essential oils?

Replacement for Prescription Drugs

One practical benefit for using essential oils is, of course, their substitutive nature; they can replace Rx drugs, which is the ultimate reason to educate yourself on their administration and to begin stockpiling your essential oil supply. One of the potential threats of economic or social collapse is the lack of resources, and primarily the inability to procure prescription drugs. Being as such, finding suitable supplements should be a priority when preparing for the worst.

Their portability is also a major bonus when it comes to survival prepping. The fact that these ultra-concentrated oils take up little-to-no space makes toting them to your shelter all the simpler should the need arise. And, because essential oils are highly concentrated, the application used in most methods of administration requires only a drop or two of oil, which means that tiny bottle will be long-lasting.

Cheap, but Effective supplement

Though money may be the last thing on your mind when it comes to prepping for a survival situation (money may even be obsolete in the event of social collapse), it is worth noting that the expense of essential oils pales in comparison to prescription drugs. In fact, whether or not you are forced to survive on essential oils due to a lack of prescription reserves, in some cases, you might consider substituting your prescriptions for these inexpensive supplements regardless. Essential oils are a cheap, but equally effective supplement to prescription medicine.

No Expiration Date

Another benefit of essential oils is that they do not expire, neither do they have "proper storage" requirements. A number of medicines and therapeutic products must be replaced every couple years, so this sets essential oils ahead of the pack when it comes to shelf life.

Versatility

Essential oils also offer great versatility. Apart from providing wellness benefits, essential oils can be repurposed for household and hygienic applications. For instance, if you're looking for something that might serve your dental hygiene needs in a time of crisis, thieves oil is your go-to essential oil. If you want to maintain your skin's wellness, frankincense and lavender will do the trick; the latter also serves as sunscreen, so you can alleviate sun damage as well.

When it comes to the house or shelter, you can use essential oils to deodorize, which will come in handy in a disaster scenario where things might start to smell fishy due to lack of proper utilities and care. For example, after the 2011 tsunami and the subsequent nuclear reactor meltdown in Japan, a nurse named Risa Nakahira used essential oils to deodorize and sanitize putrid public bathrooms in overpopulated evacuation facilities. As relief workers searched for survivors, often wading through debris and decay, Nakahira also deodorized their boots and masks using essential oils. The possibilities of these natural oils are endless.

They are also versatile when it comes to the range of patients they're capable of supporting. The wellness of everyone from your great grandfather to your infant baby can be fortified with the aid of essential oils in the appropriate dosage. They even come in handy when treating livestock or pets. From teething infants to dementia in the elderly, from teenagers with acne to dogs with urinary tract infections, essential oils can serve any patient with nearly any ailment.

Conclusion

Now that you know all about what basil essential oil can do for you – where it originates, how it's extracted, its benefits and properties, and the different methods of administration – you can use it confidently to support the body's defenses against wellness issues and start to assemble a kit of essential oils for survival. Essential oils can be purchased online or at your local holistic treatment store.

The various benefits of essential oils and their properties are countless. To build your own kit, first focus on acquiring the essential oils which may bear more relevance to your wellness issues or the potential wellness threats within your environment. In the event of a viral outbreak, for instance, basil essential oil will be one of your more crucial oils – along with oregano, lemon, frankincense and cinnamon (eBooks also available for purchase) – due to their antiviral and immuno-supportive properties.

Used as a supplement or as your go-to for digestive issues, viral infections or respiratory infections, the application of basil essential oil in medicine has survived for centuries and will survive centuries more. When it comes down to it, you don't need to rely on pharmaceuticals; essential oils, herbs, and plenty of other natural ingredients can be used to help support the body's natural defenses against any number of wellness issues, whether ailment or injury.

Essential oils are essential to your survival in the case of viral outbreak, social collapse or natural disaster because, when the SHTF, your access to pharmaceuticals will likely either be limited or eliminated altogether. supplements to our modern-day standard will equate survival when no other option exists. And when it comes to a life-or-death situation, you can't let your wellness decline, no matter the state of the world.

DISCLAIMER AND/OR LEGAL NOTICES: Every effort has been made to accurately represent this book and it's potential. Results vary with every individual, and your results may or may not be different from those depicted. No promises, guarantees or warranties, whether stated or implied, have been made that you will produce any specific result from this book. Your efforts are individual and unique, and may vary from those shown. Your success depends on your efforts, background and motivation.

The material in this publication is provided for educational and informational purposes only and is not intended as medical advice. The information contained in this book should not be used to diagnose or treat any illness, metabolic disorder, disease or health problem. Always consult your physician or healthcare provider before beginning any nutrition or exercise program. Use of the programs, advice, and information contained in this book is at the sole choice and risk of the reader.

www.ingramcontent.com/pod-product-compliance
Lightning Source LLC
Chambersburg PA
CBHW062101280526
45788CB00003B/1300